South Beach Diet

Beginners Guide to the South Beach Diet—How to Effectively Lose Weight, Feel Great and Healthy with the South Beach Diet: Including quick and easy recipes

Table of Contents

Introduction

Congratulations on downloading *South Beach Diet: Beginners Guide to the South Beach Diet—How to Effectively Lose Weight, Feel Great and Healthy with the South Beach Diet* and thank you for doing so.

The following chapters will discuss some of the basics that you should know if you would like to get started with the South Beach Diet. Many people who have gone on this diet plan have gone on other ones in the past and find that none of them work as they promise. They want something that will work, something they can stick with for the long time, and maybe something that is a bit drastic to help them lose the weight. For some, the South Beach Diet may seem a little strict, but it is meant to train the body to know what foods are good and which ones are bad in a safe and wholesome way.

In this guidebook, we are going to spend some time talking about the South Beach Diet and what it all entails. We will talk about the foods that you are allowed to eat during the different phases (this diet plan is composed of three different phases, two of which to work with losing weight and the last one to help you maintain that weight loss) and any other information that you need during these stages. We will also provide you with 40 recipes, split up into the 3 different phases, that will help you to stick through this during any phase you are in while still eating delicious foods.

When you are tired of other diet plans just not working for you and you want to finally see some of the success that you have been working so hard for, make sure to check out this guidebook and learn everything that you need about the South Beach Diet and all the great recipes that go with it!

There are plenty of books on this subject on the market, thanks again for choosing this one! Every effort was made to ensure it is full of as much useful information as possible, please enjoy!

Chapter 1: What is the South Beach Diet?

There are many different types of diets that you are able to go on during your life. Many of them are going to promise to help you lose weight and feel great, but most of them will leave you feeling like you failed in some way. Some are gong to be too restrictive and make you just drink juices or something else that is equally unhealthy all of the time. Others are going to make you concentrate on eating the wrong kinds of foods and then you will just see weight gain or other issues. None of them are going to work like you will find in the South Beach Diet.

This diet is one that is meant to help you to stay safe while losing weight quickly. While there are some diets out there that encourage you to skip meals and not eat enough calories, all three of the phases on this diet plan, even Phase 1 that is seen as the most restrictive and hardest to follow, will allow you to eat three meals each day and they all include two snacks as well. Your only requirement is to cut out the certain foods in each section and to eat until you feel pleasantly full. You won't have to skip out on snacks or meals unless you are too hungry for them.

The portions of food that you eat (and this is real and good food), will help you to get all the nutrients that you need. You will get high fiber carbs in the form of unsaturated fats, protein sources that are lean, dairy that is low fat, vegetables, whole grains, and fruits that are so good for you. Even in the first phase, you are allowed to have a little dessert to make things easier, as long as you make the right choices with this. After finishing your first two weeks on this diet plan, you will be able to even add on some red wine on occasion to the diet plan.

The goals that the South Beach Diet has include helping you to not only lose the weight in a safe and effective manner, but to help you stay fit and healthy for the rest of your life. this is not something that you can do if you go around feeling starved or tired all the time or when you are eating all the wrong foods that just add on more weight.

Yes, there are some critics to this diet who think it is too restrictive for you to follow, but there has to be some changes in the way that you eat if you would like to see changes in your weight. Too many times we take it easy on ourselves when it comes to picking out the diet plan or the foods we can eat, and this is why the weight is still there. We need to have the first phase of this diet plan, and even some of the restrictiveness of the second phase, to help us to understand the good foods we are allowed to eat so that when we do indulge, we don't go too overboard.

Now, there are three distinct phases of the South Beach Diet. The first two are meant to help with the weight loss part and the third phase is more of a maintenance to happen after you have lost all of the weight. All of these are going to work together to help you to become fit and healthy and you are able to go back to any of the phases that you would like if you start to see a backwards trend in your weight again. Keep in mind that all of these also have different rules for the kinds of foods that you are allowed to consume on them so be careful with this part. Let's take a look these different phases so we have a better understanding of how you would work with each one.

Phase 1:

When you are ready to begin on this particular diet plan, you are going to enter into Phase 1. This is the shortest phase out of all of them, but it is also one of the most restrictive in terms of what you are allowed to eat. Luckily, this one is going to be for only 2 weeks, but it is meant to help stop the cravings and to really teach the body what it is allowed to have and not have. Those who go on the South Beach Diet with a lot of weight to lose will notice that they will have a lot of cravings for refined starches and sugary foods during this part, but you will just need to hold off on those during this time.

This phase is helping you to not only get a great start with losing some of that weight, but it makes the levels of sugars in the blood more stable so that you can minimize your cravings later on. You are going to spend your time eating healthy and lean protein, such as turkey, chicken, shellfish, and fish, lots of vegetables, and nuts, low fat dairy, eggs, good fats, and so on.

During this phase, you will not feel deprived other than the cravings that may sneak up, but these are not harmful to your health. You are allowed to have three meals each day along with two snacks, and it is fine to have a dessert. But you will not be able to eat any sugars (even the sugars that are found inside of fruits) nor will you be allowed to eat any starches such as rice, pasta, and bread.

This stage is going to seem really hard at first. Your body is going to have a lot of cravings as you get rid of all those starches and sugars out of the body, and it will seem impossible. But if you are planning out your meals correctly, you should not feel hungry at all until it is time to get for another meal. If it gets hard, just remember that the first phase is only going to last for two weeks and then you are allowed to add quite a few of these foods back into the diet.

Another thing that you should remember, in addition to which foods you are allowed to eat and which ones you should avoid, is that exercise is important to this phase as well as the other phases. It is going to improve a lot of different parts of your health and will make it easier to see some of the results that you want.

During Phase 1, you are going to see that the weight loss is happening pretty rapidly, which gives a lot of positive reinforcement for this diet plan and can help you to stick with it if you can get over the cravings. When you are done, you will have gotten rid of some of the cravings and can even stabilize your blood sugars a bit better. This will make it easier when you go into the second phase because you will be better able to control the foods that you eat when some of them are reintroduced into the diet.

Phase 2:

In some cases, you will be able to get started right out with Phase 2 when you go on the South Beach Diet. If you are only trying to lose 10 pounds or less on this diet, you aren't someone who has to deal with cravings all the time, or you are just doing this as a way to improve your health, you can skip right to phase 2. For those who started with Phase 1 and then moved into Phase2, you are going to notice that you will keep going with a steady weight loss, but it will slow down. You should also notice that a lot of the cravings that you had in the past will subside.

This is the phase where you will be able to add in a lot more of the foods that were taken away during Phase 1 since now you are able to control the cravings a bit better than before. Some of the foods that you are able to include in the diet now that you are in Phase 2 include good carbs such as whole fruits, whole wheat pasta and breads, and some of the root vegetables. On some occasions, you will be able to add in a glass of white or red wine to your meal.

Remember that the weight loss is going to be slower during this period because the diet is not as restrictive at this point. This can sometimes be discouraging to people who were excited about the quick weight loss they were going through. The goal here is to get to a healthy weight that you are able to maintain with your good eating and lifestyle habits for the long term and losing weight quickly isn't something that any of us are able to handle for too long.

This is the phase that is going to help you to stay on the diet rather than see it as a quick fix. You are going to stay within phase 2 until you reach your goal weight or the weight that you are happy with. This means that the length of time that you spend in this phase is going to vary between people. Some just have a few pounds to lose and will be able to get out of this one quickly and others could spend months here working to get the weight off. Go at the pace that is right for you and keep in mind that it does take a lot longer for those who have more weight to lose.

If you do feel that you are hitting a plateau in this stage and you still have quite a bit of weight to lose, consider going back to phase 1 for a week or two to help get it kick started again.

Phase 3:

And finally you are going to get into Phase 3. This is the one that you are going to enter when you finally reach the healthy weight for you. The guidelines that are in Phase 3 are the same that other healthy Americans should follow, even those who have never had to deal with their weight. If you followed the other two phases of this diet the right way, you should now know how to make some good choices when it comes to the meals that you can consume and you will be able to take choices from any of the food groups and still stay healthy.

During this phase, you are allowed to eat from any food group, but you still need to behave and not go overboard. Sure you can have a cookie or something sweet, but stick with one and keep the rest of the meals as healthy as possible to avoid issues with gaining the weight back. If you dedicated your time to learning how to do the South Beach Diet right, you should be able to have these little cheats without having to worry about losing out the whole way.

Remember that during this process, you are allowed to go back through the phases if you would like at any time. If you are on Phase 3 for some time and feel like your eating habits are getting out of hand again or you have a big event that you would like to lose a few more pounds for, it is possible to spend some time back in Phase 1 or Phase 2 again to help out. While you should be able to stay with Phase 3 for the rest of your life and not gain weight if you do it right, there are always times when life gets in the way and the pounds may sneak back on again. Rather than letting it get out of hand, you can just re-enter a Phase of this diet from before and get things back on track.

The South Beach Diet is meant to help you learn how to work with your body and eat the foods that are good for you. It isn't going to tell you that one food is bad and one is good, but it is going to teach you that some of the foods that you are consuming on a daily basis, especially when you eat them in high amounts, are the reason that you are feeling hungry all the time while gaining weight. When you go through the phases of the South Beach Diet, you take away all of these bad foods that are causing the weight gain and then slowly add them back in so that you learn what is allowed in the body and what you are able to handle. You should be able to make good decisions for your health by the time you get to the third phase so that you can keep the weight off, even if you have a little cheat on occasion.

Chapter 2: The Truth About Carbs in the Body

When it comes to most of the diet plans that you have tried in the past, there is one thing that most of them will have in common. Most of these are going to tell you that fat is the enemy, that these fats are the things that are making you sick and making it hard to lose weight. If you are able to reduce the amount of fats that you are eating, you will be able to lose weight.

There are a number of problems with this though. The first issue is that these diets see that there are differences between bad fats and good fats. There is a difference when it comes to the type of fats that you eat. If you are eating saturated fats from your favorite fast food restaurant each day, you are going to get sick and have all the issues that those other diet plans promise. But there are plenty of healthy fats that you can consume, ones that come in healthy protein sources and fish that will fuel the body, help the mind, and just make you feel better overall. If you miss out on some of these healthy fats, you are going to end up causing a lot of harm to the body because it is missing out on some important nutrients that it needs.

The next issue is what you are replacing these fats with. Since you aren't getting your nutrition from the healthy fats that the body needs, you are going to need to get them from somewhere. Most of these diets ask you to get the nutrition from carbs. But just like with fats, there are good carbs and bad carbs and these are not distinguished from in these diet plans either.

When you consume carbs, especially since most people are going to choose the bad carbs instead of the good ones, you are consuming a really unhealthy form of energy. Your body is not going to be able to process this properly, which is why you feel that burst of energy in the beginning and then go through a big crash shortly after. This is because the carbs that you are consuming are being converted into sugars inside the body, sugars that you aren't using up as quickly as you should and which can make you feel sick, worn down, and add to belly fat in no time.

These diets have been telling it to you wrong for so long now. You are eating the wrong kind of nutrition into your diet each day, taking in the harmful carbs that are adding to excess fat around the body and raising your blood sugars to abnormal heights. You need those good fats in your life if you would like to be healthy, but too many times we are told that all fats are bad, so we learn how to stay away from them.

Fats are better for the body. They are the most efficient form of energy for the body possible. When you bring these into the body, you are not converting them into something that is hard on the body (such as carbs that will turn into sugars and not be used). You are bringing in something that will provide you with energy all day long. Some people do notice a lag in their energy levels right at the beginning, but this is mostly because the body is looking for carbs and it takes it a bit to learn to rely on the fat stores instead.

But there are going to be some pretty amazing things that happen when you start to reduce the amount of carbs that you are consuming in favor of more fats. First, you are going to have more energy because the fat is able to keep the body going for a much longer time. The body is going to see the fat that you are consuming and just eat it up, helping you to feel ready to take on the day. And then, when the body is done using the fat that you consume, it is going to turn around and start eating up the fat that is stored all around your body. Once the body starts to use fats instead of carbs as the main source of energy, you will be able to see it eat through the body fat without any extra work!

Another benefit is that foods that are full of the healthy fats are the ones that will fill you up for much longer. Think back to those diets that you were on in the past; where there many days that you just felt hungry all the time, no matter how many calories you took in? This is most likely because you aren't taking in any of the fats that you need, the ones that fill you up and make you feel full and satisfied after a meal.

While on the South Beach Diet, you are going to learn to control the amount of carbs that you are eating, especially during the first two phases. This diet doesn't assume that all carbs are bad (there are plenty of carbs that can be good and provide good nutrition), but it recognizes that most of us don't know how to determine good carbs from bad and most of us eat way too much of them. We need to learn how to monitor the carbs that we are eating and so we take most of them away, and focus instead on some of the healthy fats and other foods that we are allowed to eat on this diet plan.

There are still plenty of great meals that you will be able to enjoy when you are on this kind of diet plan, but you will have to shift the focus that you are eating with in order to see the best results. The good news is that these high fat meals are going to taste good and be filling, so you will eat fewer calories, without feeling deprived, and still be able to lose weight all at the same time.

The South Beach Diet is the perfect way to help you to work with the carbs that are in your body. On your typical American diet, you are spending a lot of time consuming the carbs that you just don't need. You are taking in large amounts of baked goods, pizzas, breads, and other things. And when the cravings come around, it is hard to say no and just stay away from them. But the South Beach Diet is going to help.

It is important to realize that the South Beach Diet is not against carbs. This diet plan realizes that there is some importance to the carbs in your diet, but it is trying to help you to learn what carbs are good and in what amounts you should be eating those carbs. Yes, the first phase of the diet is going to pretty much eliminate the carbs as much as possible, but this is not because all carbs are bad; it is simply a way to help you quickly get through the issues you have with cravings. Once you get past that first two-week period, you can slowly add in those carbs and when you get to the third phase, you can eat any carbs that you would like as long as you do so in moderation and you are careful to eat the ones that are whole wheat or whole grain.

While this diet plan is going to seem hard in the beginning, especially when those cravings start to come and bug you, you will find that it is the fastest and safest way to get rid of those cravings so that you can make informed and healthy choices about the carbs that you consume. Most of this diet is going to focus on the healthy produce and the healthy fats that you can consume, but if you learn how to get rid of the cravings and instead go for the good carbs that are going to fill you up (mainly whole wheat and plenty of produce), you are allowed to have some carbs on this diet plan.

So what are you going to eat when you are on the South Beach Diet? We just talked about how you will need to limit your carb intake on the first two phases of this diet, but what is there left to eat. When you are on the first phase, you are going to concentrate on healthy fats and proteins, such as lean turkey and chicken and lots of fish. You can have a few vegetables, but you will concentrate more on the low fat dairy, the protein, and the healthy oils.

Then on the second phase, you are able to add in more of the carbs if you would like. This is going to include healthy carbs though and you will want to go pretty slowly to get started. For example, maybe start the first week with an extra serving of vegetables and then move in to having some fruits in there and finally get to adding in the carbs, once you know that your carvings are better under control.

The second phase can last some time depending on how much weight you are trying to lose, but when you get to the third phase, you will be able to enjoy any of the carbs you would like, as long as you are taking them in moderation. This means you can have that snack or dessert on occasion, you just need to be smart about it. By this point you should know more about your body and what it is allowed to have and how to avoid the cravings so indulging on occasion is not going to be such a bad thing.

While the other diets are going to keep telling you that the fats are bad and the carbs are good, you will see that they just don't have the success that you are used to when working with this great diet plan.

Chapter 3: The 3 Phases in South Beach Diet and Foods Allowed in Each One

There are three phases that are recognized on the South Beach Diet. Each of these are meant to help you to lose weight and learn how to properly eat different foods in your life. The first phase is going to be the most restrictive when it comes to the foods that are allowed, but you will find that all of the phases have some rules about food so that you learn how to properly eat for weight loss and weight loss maintenance.

The Phase 1 Foods

The first phase is one of the most important parts of the South Beach Diet, even though it is only going to last for two weeks. This phase is going to help you to go from your old habits to healthier ones that are allowed on this diet plan. Most Americans are used to taking in a lot of unhealthy carbs ad foods and eating way too much of them. This means that they are going to take on foods that are making them gain weight and not feel good. During the first phase, we are going to eliminate a lot of the foods that are causing the weight gain and the bad cravings so that we can break the cycle and learn how to eat in a much healthier way.

The first phase is one of the hardest ones. This is the diet plan that is trying to make sure that you get rid of some of the cravings that are driving you insane and making it hard to give up your foods. But these cravings are going to be hard to fight so you need to be ready to give them up. You are only going to be allowed a few carbs (like half a cup of vegetables a day) in this phase in order to finally break up the amount of cravings that you are dealing with on a daily basis.

So on this part of the diet, you will be limiting a lot of the foods that you are allowed to eat. But the important part to remember here is that it is for your good health. This phase is hard, but it only lasts you for two weeks before moving on to the second phase and then you are allowed to bring a lot of these carbs back in the second phase after the cravings.

First, let's talk about the meats that you are allowed to eat on the first phase. There are many great meat sources that you are allowed to eat, you just need to make sure that you are not eating the ones that have been processed and can make you feel really sick with all the sugars and carbs that are added in. Some of the meat options that you are able to enjoy include turkey and Canadian bacon, chicken breast, turkey, lean cuts of beef, boiled ham, lunch meats that are lower in fat, seafood of all kinds, and even soy based meat substitutes.

If you are not a fan of meat or you are a vegetarian, you are able to use many types of beans to ensure that you are able to find the right amount of protein to make you feel good. Some of the most popular forms of beans that you are allowed to eat on this diet include pinto beans, chickpeas, great northern beans, and black eyed peas.

Nuts are another part of the South Beach Diet that you are allowed to consume and enjoy. You will need to limit the serving to just one each day. This is enough to allow you to get all the good nutrients that you need out of the nuts, but still makes sure that you don't take in too many that will make you feel overwhelmed with too much fat.

There are some limits on the types of vegetables that you are allowed to consume. Most of them are going to be fine, but there are a lot that have more carbs in them than you are allowed on this part of the diet. You will be able to add them back in later on but this phase is going to restrict them a little bit. Remember that since you are restricting your carbs on this part that you are only allowed to have about half a cup of these to stay healthy and to beat the cravings. Some of the vegetables that you can have on this part of the diet plan include peppers, Brussels Sprouts, Broccoli, Cauliflower, okra, spinach, sprouts, lettuce, mushrooms, onions, squash, and tomatoes.

In addition, you are allowed to have some dairy and fats in order to stay full and happy on this part of the diet plan. It is common to eat cheeses that are low in fat, salad dressing that is low in sugar (and only a few tablespoons of this each day), avocado, a few tablespoons of a healthy oil, egg whites and whole eggs, and cottage cheese.

You may notice on this section that you are not allowed to have any fruits. These are high in carbs and are not the healthiest option. Most fruits are considered healthy of course, but while you are going through this part of the diet and working to get through the cravings that are making you unhealthy, you will need to refrain from eating fruits for now. The good news is that you will be able to add them back in later on.

These are the major food groups that you need to focus on when you are trying to get started on the South Beach Diet. It is restrictive, but you are going to notice that your cravings get smaller and smaller as you go through the two weeks and you will notice that you can lose a good amount of weight on this phase of the diet plan too, making it easier to find enough encouragement to keep on going through these two weeks.

The Phase 2 Foods

After you get done with the first phase of the South Beach Diet (thank goodness after all that hard work and missing out on some of your favorite foods!) it is time to move on to the second phase. This one is still going to have some restrictions, but it is also going to help allow a few more things back on. You will be able to have some fruits again for example. But remember that you still need to be a bit limiting on what you are allowed to consume so that you are still able to lose the weight during this time.

During this phase, you will be allowed to eat the same foods as the first phase, but you can also start to reintroduce some more foods to the diet. You should go slowly though. It is not a good idea to flood the body with carbs, even good carbs that are found inside of fruits and vegetables, because this is going to trigger the cravings to come back and can make it so you need to re-enter phase 1 again. You should slowly add in some healthy carbs to the diet, but do it slowly and a little bit at a time.

You may feel that adding in a serving a day for a week may be a good idea. Then you can get a few more that you were supposed to be avoiding, but you still aren't overdoing it either. Perhaps start out by adding in some more fruits and vegetables to start for a few weeks, such as for treats so that your body gets used to the healthy carbs first. Once you are done with this part, you can start to add in some of the other carbs, such as whole grain pastas and whole grain breads, as long as you go slowly and add them in without flooding the system.

During this phase, you will also want to be careful with not taking in too much bread. This is the phase where you are allowed to eat some products that are whole grain and some brown rice, but you do need to be careful. There is a lot of marketing that promises the product is how you want, but when you look at the ingredients, you will find that this is false. You should always check the label and make sure that it has at least 3g or more of fiber in each serving and that it has not been processed.

In addition, you are allowed to add in some alcohol, as long as you do this in moderation. You are not allowed to go out and party each night and say it is part of the South Beach Diet. But if you have a glass of wine with supper, you are able to get some heart benefits with your meal. But taking in more than this can cause more harm than good, especially with all the carbs that you are taking in, and you don't want this.

This is a phase where you should take some time to equip the kitchen in order to get it ready for some healthy living for the rest of your life. Remember that the South Beach Diet is all about finding healthy ways to keep on it for the rest of your life. This is not a fad diet that you go on for a few months and then give up. There are two weight loss phases and then one that is meant to help you to maintain that weight loss for years to come. But one of the steps for you to do this is to make sure that your kitchen is ready to help.

A good place to start is with a scale. This helps you to measure out how much of each food you are consuming so you don't go overboard with the carbs. For example, fruits are really easy to overeat so having a scale around to help you measure it all out can help. Measuring cups, approved food lists, and even making sure to clean out the pantry and only have good foods around can all help you to succeed.

And finally, learning how to eat with mindfulness is important when it comes to being healthy. Most of us overeat because we spend time in front of the television eating, we eat in the car, we scarf down the meal without thinking and so much else. We eat because we are bored or sad or because it is convenient, not because we are hungry.

On the South Beach Diet, you don't need to count the calories as much, but you do need to practice mindful eating. You need to eat when the body is hungry, rather than when you are bored or sad. You need to sit down and enjoy your meals, rather than hurrying through them and eating as much as possible. Taking slow and deliberate bites, prolonging the meal, and just enjoying yourself can really help to make it easier to eat the right amount, while still feeling full, on this diet plan.

During Phase 2, you are still working on losing the weight and feeling good, but you will see that there are still some restrictions on what you are allowed to eat. In addition, the weight loss is going to slow way down. You may lose five to ten pounds in the first few weeks on the South Beach Diet because of all the foods that you are getting rid of and the fact that the body is taking in fewer calories. But things kind of even out on the second phase and you are more likely to lose between 1 and 2 pounds a week instead. You will stick with this phase until you reach your weight loss goals, with perhaps a quick visit back to Phase 1 if you get stuck or need some extra help.

The Phase 3 Foods

When you get to Phase 3, you should be able to add in most of the foods that you had to take out before. This makes it easier for you to eat more of a variety in your diet without being as restrictive as you had to be in some of the other options. You will still need to be careful in this one though. You need to remember that while you are allowed to have a few cheats here and there because you should know how to eat properly for your body by this point, that it can be easy to fall back into old habits and take more calories than you want.

If you stick with what you learned in the South Beach Diet and don't go overboard, you are able to add in all the foods back to your diet. You can have a cheat day with a cookie or another sweet, as long as you keep it in moderation. You should concentrate your efforts on eating healthy and whole foods like fruits, lean meats, whole grains, vegetables, nuts, and dairy that is low in fat and seeds instead of the bad stuff though, even on this part of the diet. You most likely won't be losing weight on this section though since this is more of the maintenance phase of the diet instead of the weight loss part, but you still need to continue to eat the good foods that your body needs to stay healthy.

When it comes to the different phases that are needed in this diet plan, you need to make sure that you are eating the right kinds of foods. Each of these phases is important to help you to really lose the weight and feel good. The different phases are important because they all help you in different ways on this journey to help you to lose weight and feel good.

Chapter 4: Recipes During Phase 1 of the South Beach Diet

Vegetable Hash

Ingredients:

Minced garlic clove (1)
Diced zucchini (2)
Chopped mushrooms (4)
Diced red bell pepper (1)
Salt
Paprika
Thyme
Chopped onion (1)
Olive oil (1 Tbsp.)

Directions:

1. Bring out a skillet and heat some oil on it. When this is warm, add the thyme, onion, and paprika.
2. Reduce the heat a bit and then stir this for 7 minutes so the onion can become soft.
3. Now add in the garlic, zucchini, mushrooms, bell pepper, and salt. Cover the skillet and let it stir for another 4 minutes.
4. Take off the heat and serve.

Quiche Cups

Ingredients:

Diced onion (1/4 c.)
Green bell pepper (1/4 c.)
Hot pepper sauce (3 drops)
Egg substitute (3/4 c.)
Cheddar cheese (3/4 c.)
Chopped spinach (1 pkg.)

Directions:

1. Turn on the oven to preheat to 350 degrees. Take out a muffin pan and spray with some cooking spray.
2. Place the spinach into a container and cook for 2 ½ minutes. Drain out any liquid that is extra.
3. Bring out a big bowl and combine together the pepper sauce, onion, bell pepper, egg substitute, cheese, and spinach.
4. Mix this well and divide the mixture between the muffin cups. Place into the oven and let it cook for 20 minutes.

Green Gazpacho

Ingredients:

Olive oil (1 Tbsp.)
Water (2 Tbsp.)
Cayenne (1/8 tsp.)
Lime juice (2 Tbsp.)
Peeled garlic clove (1)
Chopped scallions (2)
Chopped green bell pepper (1)
Chopped lettuce, red leaf (2 c.)
Chopped cucumber (2 ½ lbs.)
Diced avocado (1)
Salt (1/4 tsp.)

Directions:

1. Take out a blender and puree the cumin, salt, oil, water, lime juice, garlic, scallions, pepper, lettuce, and cucumbers. Season with some more salt if needed.
2. Move this to a big bowl. Let this chill for a minimum of 2 hours, but overnight is better.
3. When it is time to serve, peel and dice up the avocado and divide this between 4 bowls before adding the avocado and serving.

Tomato Soup

Ingredients:

White mushrooms (5 oz.)
Red pepper flakes (1/4 tsp.)
Basil (1/4 tsp.)
Oregano (1/4 tsp.)
Minced garlic cloves (4)
Minced celery stalks (2)
Minced onion (1)
Olive oil (1 Tbsp.)
Water (3/4 c.)
Tomato sauce (1 can)
Lima beans (1 can)
Diced tomatoes (1 can)
Diced summer squash (1)

Directions:

1. Bring out a pan and heat some oil on it. Add the pepper flakes, oregano, basil, garlic, celery, and onion.
2. Cook this for 5 minutes. Add in the mushrooms and squash. Let these bake a bit longer.
3. Add in the tomatoes and their juices along with the diced tomatoes and beans. Bring this to a simmer.
4. Continue to cook until everything is heated through and then serve.

White Bean Soup

Ingredients:

Northern beans (1 can)
Salt
Thyme
Rosemary (1/2 tsp.)
Garlic cloves (2)
Basil (1/2 tsp.)
Chopped celery stalk (1)
Chopped onion (1)

Olive oil (1)
Vegetable broth (1 ½ c.)

Directions:

1. Bring out a pan and heat it up with the oil inside. Add the salt, thyme, rosemary, basil, garlic, celery, and onion. Let the heat come down a bit and cook a little longer.
2. When the vegetables are soft, add in the beans and stir. After this is warm, move ¾ of the mixture to a blender and add the broth.
3. Puree this until smooth and then return to the pan. Bring this to a simmer to make warm and then season with some pepper and salt to taste.

Labne Balls

Ingredients:

Olive oil
Italian seasoning (2 Tbsp.)
Salt (1 tsp.)
Greek yogurt (3 containers)

Directions:

1. Take out a strainer and line it with a cheesecloth. Place this over a bowl. Bring out a second bowl and combine the salt and yogurt.
2. Spoon this all into the strainer and then cover with the plastic wrap. Let this set in the fridge for 48 hours. You will notice that you have 1 ½ cups of drained yogurt after this time.
3. Place the Italian seasonings in a dish. Take out a piece of waxed paper and then roll out the yogurt into small balls. Roll these through the Italian seasonings.
4. Serve these right away.

Skillet Cod

Ingredients:

Cod fillets (4)
Peguillo peppers (2)
Drained diced tomatoes (1 can)
Pepper
Salt
Minced garlic cloves (3)
Sliced onion (1)
Sliced zucchini (1)
Olive oil (1 Tbsp.)
Parsley (2 Tbsp.)

Directions:

1. Take out a big skillet and heat some oil. Add the pepper, salt, garlic, onion, and zucchini, letting it cook for 10 minutes.
2. Now add in the peppers and tomatoes and let it heat for 10 more minutes.
3. Add the fish into the sauce, making sure to add some to the top. Cover this and let the fish cook until it is opaque, which will take around 10 minutes.
4. Sprinkle on a bit of parsley and then serve warm.

Tomato and Spinach Salmon

Ingredients:

Baby spinach (3 c.)
Chopped tomatoes (1 lb.)
Minced garlic cloves (2)
Chopped onion (1)
Olive oil (1 Tbsp.)
Pepper
Salt
Salmon fillets (4)
Lemon wedges (4)
Drained capers (1 Tbsp.)

Directions:

1. Heat up the oven to be at broil. Use some cooking spray to prepare a baking dish.
2. Place the salmon into the baking dish and season with pepper and salt. Add this to the baking dish.
3. Broil the salmon for 10 minutes to cook through, but don't turn it.
4. While the salmon is broiling, bring out your skillet and let the oil cook inside a bit. Add in the onion and garlic, stirring a few times for 7 minutes. Then add in the capers, spinach, and tomatoes and cook another 2 minutes.
5. Remove the salmon from the oven and put it on 4 plates. Spoon the tomato mixture on top and squeeze a bit of lemon over it. Serve warm.

Pecan Trout

Ingredients:

Olive oil (2 tsp.)
Beaten egg (1)
Salt (1/4 tsp.)
Whole trout (4)
Cayenne (1/8 tsp.)
Garlic clove (1)
Rosemary (1 tsp.)
Pecans (1/2 c.)

Directions:

1. Heat the oven up to 400 degrees. Lay out a baking sheet and cover it with parchment paper.
2. Place the cayenne, garlic, rosemary, and pecans into the food processor and chop them until they are fine. Move this to a shallow dish.
3. Place the trout onto a baking sheet and season with salt. Brush on some egg white before sprinkling the nut mixture all over the egg whites and pressing down.
4. Drizzle with some oil and bake the trout for 20 minutes to cook through before serving.

Ginger Tenderloin

Ingredients:

Pepper
Olive oil (1 ½ tsp.)
Sliced garlic cloves (1)
Pork loin (1 ½ lbs.)
Salt
ginger (1 tsp.)
sour cream (1 Tbsp.)
thyme
Dijon mustard (1 ½ Tbsp.)

Directions:

1. Start this recipe by turning on the oven to 450 degrees. While that heats up, bring out a bowl and stir the salt, thyme, ginger, sour cream, and mustard together.
2. Make small slits in the pork loin and then slip the garlic into the slits. Brush with the oil and add some pepper and salt.
3. Heat up a skillet on the stove. Add the pork loin and let it brown on all of the sides.
4. Now add on the mustard mixture and then move the pan you are working with over to your oven. Leave it inside the oven for a bit so the pork can cook through.
5. Give this some time to cool after done with the oven and slice the pork a bit before serving.

Shepherd's Pie

Ingredients:

Pepper
Worcestershire sauce (2 tsp.)
Beef broth (1/2 c.)
Shelled edamame (2 c.)
Beef (1 lb.)
Minced garlic cloves (2)
Chopped onion (1)

Olive oil (1 Tbsp.)
Cauliflower florets (1 pkg.)
Salt
Cheddar cheese (1/2 c.)
Egg yolk (1)
Sour cream (2 Tbsp.)

Directions:

1. Heat up the oven to 350 degrees. Fill up you're pot with a bit of water. Throw in the cauliflower and allow it to boil for a bit to become soft. Drain out.
2. In a skillet, heat up some oil before cooking the garlic and onion inside for 5 minutes. Take the beef and add it to a big skillet. Allow it to cook until the lumps are gone and the beef is brown.
3. Take the edamame and throw in with the beef to cook. Stir the broth, pepper, salt, and Worcestershire sauce in as well. Move this over to the baking dish.
4. Use an electric mixer and whip the cauliflower with the salt, egg yolk, and sour cream. Spoon this on top of the meat and then top with some cheese.
5. Bake for 25 minutes and then serve warm.

Veggie Chili

Ingredients:

Pinto beans (2 cans)
Salt
Cumin (1 tsp.)
Oregano (1 Tbsp.)
Chili powder (1 Tbsp.)
Minced garlic cloves
Chopped celery stalks (2)
Chopped onion (1)
Chopped mushrooms (1 ½ c.)
Bell peppers (2)
Olive oil (1 Tbsp.)
Diced tomatoes (1 can)

Directions:

1. Bring out a pan and heat some oil on high. Add the garlic, celery, pepper, onion, and mushrooms
2. Cook these together to help the vegetables to soften. Then add in the salt, cumin, oregano, and chili powder.
3. Allow these to cook for another 5 minutes. Add in the tomatoes and the beans and bring all of this to a simmer.
4. Allow the chili to cook for another 30 minutes before serving.

Potato Salad

Ingredients:

Pepper
Chives (2 Tbsp.)
Hearts of palm (2 cans)
Olive oil (1 Tbsp.)
Minced garlic clove (1)
Dijon mustard (1 tsp.)
Lemon juice (2 tsp.)

Directions:

1. Bring out a big bowl and whisk together the lemon juice, garlic, and mustard. While whisking, add in the oil a bit at a time.
2. Then add in the chives and the hearts of palm. Toss it all around to combine.
3. Season with a bit of pepper before serving.

Red Bean Mash

Ingredients:

Pepper
Cilantro (3 Tbsp.)
Salt (1/4 tsp.)
Vegetable broth (1/2 c.)
Red kidney beans (1 can)

Minced garlic cloves (3)
Chopped onion (1)
Olive oil (1 Tbsp.)

Directions:

1. Bring out a pan and heat some oil. Add in the garlic and onion and let these cook until they are soft which takes 7 minutes.
2. Add in the salt, broth, and beans and then bring to a simmer. Cook for another 5 minutes.
3. Take the pan off the heat and stir in the cilantro. Use a potato masher to mash this into a puree.
4. Add some pepper and then serve warm.

Baked Ricotta Custard

Ingredients:

Cinnamon
Vanilla (1/4 tsp.)
Half and half (1/4 c.)
Egg white (1)
Egg (1)
Sugar substitute (1/4 c.)
Cream cheese (4 oz.)
Ricotta cheese (3/4 c.)

Directions:

1. Take out a bowl and use your electric mixer to beat the cream cheese and ricotta until creamy. Add in the sugar and beat until combine.
2. At this time, add in the egg, vanilla, egg white, and half and half to mix until well blended.
3. Move this mixture over to 4 prepared ramekins and then place these into a baking dish.
4. Add some hot water into the baking dish to about an inch and then place into the oven.

5. Turn the oven on to 350 degrees and let the custard cook for 45 minutes. Take out of the water bath and cool down before serving with some cinnamon.

Chapter 5: Recipes for Phase 2 of the South Beach Diet

Egg Frijoles

Ingredients:

Salsa (1 c.)
Beaten eggs (4)
Tortillas (4)
Cayenne (1/8 tsp.)
Pinto beans (2 cans)
Dried oregano (1 Tbsp.)
Minced garlic cloves (3)
Chopped onion (1)
Olive oil (1 Tbsp. and 1 ½ tsp.)

Directions:

1. Bring out a skillet and heat up some oil on it. Add on the oregano, garlic, and onion, stirring a few times to make the onion soft.
2. Add the cayenne and beans and then simmer, stirring a few times to make the beans warm and flavorful, which takes around 10 minutes. Cover and keep warm.
3. While these are cooking, warm up the tortillas. When there is a bit of time left with the beans, take out another skillet and heat up the rest of the oil. Add the eggs and scramble them for 5 minutes.
4. Divide the beans between the tortillas and top with salsa and eggs. Roll up and enjoy.

Oat Muffins

Ingredients:

Chopped walnuts (2/3 c.)
Salt (1/4 tsp.)
Cinnamon (1/4 tsp.)
Baking soda (1/2 tsp.)
Baking powder (1 ½ tsp.)

Pastry flour (1 ¼ c.)
Rolled oats (3/4 c. 2 Tbsp.)
Buttermilk (1 c.)
Vanilla (1 tsp.)
Beaten egg (1)
Canola oil (1/3 c.)
Brown sugar substitute (1/3 c.)

Directions:

1. Turn on the oven and let it heat up to 425 degrees. Prepare a few muffin pans.
2. In a bowl, combine ¾ cup of oats with the buttermilk and let it soak for at least 30 minutes.
3. In another bowl and add in the flour, baking soda, salt, baking powder, and cinnamon. Slowly add in the walnuts.
4. In another bowl, stir in the vanilla, egg, oil, and brown sugar. Slowly add in the oat mixture and then the flour mixture until they just start to combine.
5. Divide this between the muffin cups and then sprinkle the rest of the oats over the muffins.
6. Bake for 15 minutes and allow some time to cool before serving.

Eggsadilla

Ingredients:

Pepper Jack cheese (2 oz.)
Tortilla (1)
Pepper
Salt
Beaten egg (3)
Olive oil (1 tsp.)

Directions:

1. Bring out a skillet and heat up the oil. Add the eggs and then reduce to medium.
2. Scramble the eggs until they are cooked, which will take 2 minutes. Move to a plate and season a bit.

3. Wipe out the pan and add in the tortilla, cooking on each side for just a few seconds to warm through.
4. Top half the tortilla with cheese and then with eggs. Fold the other half over and cook for another minute before serving.

Thai Shrimp Soup

Ingredients:

Asian fish sauce (2 tsp.)
Chili garlic sauce (2 tsp.)
Tomatoes (2)
Shrimp (1 lb.)
Coconut milk (1 can)
Jalapeno pepper (1)
Sliced ginger (1)
Sliced scallions (2)
Lemon juice (4 Tbsp.)
Chicken broth (4 c.)

Directions:

1. Bring out a pan and combine the pepper, ginger, scallion whites, lemon juice, broth. Take this up to boiling. Then turn down the heat and simmer.
2. Stir in the coconut milk, fish sauce, garlic sauce, tomatoes, and shrimp. Return this to a simmer and cook for another 3 minutes.
3. Remove the pan off the heat and divide this between 4 bowls. Sprinkle on some scallion greens and serve.

Roasted Tomato Soup

Ingredients:

Vegetable broth (1 c.)
Olive oil (1 Tbsp.)
Pepper
Salt (1/4 tsp.)
Oregano (1 tsp.)

Basil (1 Tbsp.)
Peeled garlic cloves (4)
Diced onion (1)
Tomatoes (2 ½ lbs.)

Directions:

1. Turn on the oven and let it heat up to 425 degrees. Place some parchment paper on a baking pan. Arrange the tomatoes onto the pan and then scatter some garlic and onion on it.
2. Sprinkle on some pepper, salt, oregano, basil, and garlic. Drizzle a bit of oil on top.
3. Bake these inside the oven until the dish is done, or around 40 minutes. After this time, take the mixture out of the oven and move to a blender. Add in ½ cup of broth.
4. Puree this until it is smooth. Move this over to a pan and then stir in the rest of the broth. Bring to a simmer and let it heat up before serving.

Turkey Sausage Soup

Ingredients:

Chicken broth (3 ¼ c.)
Escarole (1 head)
Minced garlic clove (1)
Salt
Rosemary (1/2 tsp.)
Chopped onion (1)
Olive oil (1 Tbsp.)
Turkey sausage (8 oz.)

Directions:

1. Coat a saucepan with some cooking spray and then add the sausages. Reduce the heat a bit and then brown on all sides for 10 minutes. Move to a cutting board.
2. Add some oil to the pan and heat it up. Add the salt, rosemary, and onion and allow it to go six minutes.

3. Throw minutes. Cut the sausages in half going lengthwise and then into pieces.
4. Add the escarole to the pan, going in batches, and then stir to make it wilted. Add broth and sausage and bring to a simmer. Cook another two minutes and serve.

Florentine Soup

Ingredients:

Chicken broth (3 c.)
Cubed cream cheese (2 oz.)
Spinach (1 pkg.)
Chicken breasts (2)
Pepper
Salt
Sliced garlic cloves (2)
Chopped onion (1)
Olive oil (1 Tbsp.)

Directions:

1. Bring out a pan and heat the oil. Add in the pepper, salt, onion, and garlic. Allow this to cook together for seven minutes.
2. Throw the spinach and chicken and stir for a minute before adding in the cream cheese. Stir this until it is melted.
3. Now add in the broth and bring it to a simmer. Keep cooking until the chicken can cook through before serving.

Stuffed Chicken Breast

Ingredients:

Salt
Chicken breast (4)
Pepper
Basil (1/2 tsp.)
Minced garlic clove (1)

Chopped sun dried tomatoes (2)
Feta cheese (1/3 c.)
Olive oil (2 tsp.)

Directions:

1. Preheat the oven to 425 degrees. Bring out a bowl and combine the basil, garlic, tomatoes, and cheese. Season with some pepper and then mash it together with the fork.
2. Butterfly the chicken and then open up each breast and spread with some of the feta mixture.
3. Close the breast with the filling and press the edges together to seal it up. Season with some pepper and salt.
4. Bring out a skillet and heat some oil on the stove. Add in the chicken and cook to brown on both sides, about 2 minutes each.
5. Move the skillet and place inside of the oven and then just let it cook to finish up the chicken.

Chicken and Soba Noodles

Ingredients:

Vegetable oil (1 tsp.)
Sesame oil (2 tsp.)
Soy sauce (1 Tbsp.)
Salt
Red pepper flakes (1/2 tsp.)
Ginger (1 tsp.)
Sliced garlic cloves (3)
Scallions (4)
Chicken breasts (1 ½ lbs.)
Soba noodles (4 oz.)
Lemon juice (2 tsp.)
Water (2 Tbsp.)
Button mushrooms (6 oz.)
Sliced Napa cabbage (1 head)

Directions:

1. Bring out a pan and bring water to boil. Cook the noodles until the are done.
2. While this is cooking, bring out a bowl and combine together the salt, pepper flakes, ginger, garlic, scallion whites, and chicken.
3. Drain out the noodles and move over to a bowl. Add in the sesame oil, soy sauce, and scallion greens.
4. In a skillet, heat the vegetable oil. Cook the chicken for about 5 minutes and then move to a plate.
5. Now add the water, mushrooms, and cabbage. Cook until the vegetables wilt. Add the chicken back in and cook for another minute.
6. Toss with some lemon juice and serve.

Herbed Turkey

Ingredients:

Chopped parsley (4 Tbsp.)
Italian bread crumbs (1 c.)
Milk (2 Tbsp.)
Beaten egg (1)
Pepper
Salt
Minced garlic clove (3)
Turkey cutlets (1 ½ lbs.)
Button mushrooms (1 lb.)
Olive oil (1 Tbsp.)

Directions:

1. Coat the turkey with some of the garlic and salt and pepper. Bring out a small bowl and whisk the milk and egg. Spread out the bread crumbs on a big plate.
2. Dredge the turkey into the egg mixture and then through the bread crumbs on both sides.
3. Use some cooking spray to cover a skillet and cook the turkey in batches until crisp. Sprinkle with some parsley and then cover with foil to keep it warm.

4. Add the oil as well as the remainder of the garlic and parsley along with the mushrooms into your skillet. Cook for 5 minutes.
5. Move the turkey to the plates and then top with some mushrooms before serving.

Halibut and Vegetable Ragout

Ingredients:

Chopped tomatoes (2)
Pepper
Basil
Salt
Crushed garlic cloves (2)
Chopped onion (1)
Olive oil (2 tsp.)
Halibut fillet (4 pieces)
Butter beans (1 can)
Peas (1 c.)

Directions:

1. To begin this recipe, bring out a pan and heat up some oil. Add the pepper, basil, salt, garlic, and onion.
2. Reduce the heat and let it cook for 4 minutes. Stir your peas inside of this along with the tomatoes and allow it to warm up.
3. Now add in the beans and cook for another 2 minutes. Take the pan off the heat.
4. Place the halibut into a broiler pan and brush with some oil. Broil until it is opaque, which would take about 8 minutes.
5. Divide this among four plates and serve the fish and the ragout together.

Shrimp and Scallop Bake

Ingredients:

Chopped parsley (1 Tbsp.)

Lemon zest (2 tsp.)
Lemon juice (2 tsp)
Olive oil (1 Tbsp.)
Pepper
Salt
Minced garlic cloves (3)
Shrimp (3/4)
Sea scallops (3/4 lb.)

Directions:

1. To start this recipe, bring out a bowl and combine the garlic, shrimp, scallops and season with pepper. Toss this around until the seafood is coated through.
2. Bring out a skillet and heat up the oil. Add your premade seafood mixture and cook it for about 4 minutes.
3. Move over to a serving bowl and add lemon zest and juice. Sprinkle a bit of parsley and serve this warm.

Stir-fry with Beef

Ingredients:

Water (2 Tbsp.)
Snow peas (6 oz.)
Minced garlic clove (1)
Sliced onion (1)
Sliced green bell pepper (1)
Olive oil (1 tsp.)
Pepper
Round steak (1 ½ lbs.)
Soy sauce (1 Tbsp.)

Directions:

1. Take the steak with some pepper and salt. Bring out a skillet and coat with some cooking spray.
2. Add the steak inside and cook for about 4 minutes and then move off the heat. Move the steak to a board and give it 5 minutes to cool before you slice it.

3. Inside this pan, allow the oil to get warm before throwing in the pepper, garlic, and onion, cooking these for 5 minutes.
4. Add in the water and peas and cook until the vegetables are soft and let it cook for 5 minutes.
5. Uncover the pot and add in the soy sauce. Cook this for another 30 seconds. Add the sliced steak and toss it around a bit. Serve it warm.

Lamb Stew

Ingredients:

Rosemary (2 tsp.)
Peeled and smashed garlic cloves (4)
Chopped onion (1)
Celeriac (1 diced)
Diced carrots (2)
Pepper
Salt
Lamb (1 ½ lbs.)
Olive oil (3 tsp.)
Peeled tomatoes (1 can)
Dry red wine (1/3 c.)
Tomato paste (1 Tbsp.)

Directions:

1. In a pan, heat up some oil and add in the lamb. Cook for about 6 minutes so that the lamb is browned on the outside. Move this over to a plate.
2. Add in the rest of the oil to the same pan and add in the rosemary, garlic, onion, celeriac, and carrots.
3. Cook, stirring until the vegetables will start to brown. Add the tomato paste and cook another minute before adding the wine and cooking some more.
4. Add in the tomatoes and their juice before bringing this to a simmer. Allow this to be a bit cooler and cook for a bit to let everything get nice and warm.
5. Return the lamb and cook to heat it through before serving.

Barley Risotto

Ingredients:

Pepper
Salt
Parmesan cheese (1/4 c.)
Pearled barley (1/2 c.)
Sliced onion (1)
Olive oil (2 tsp.)
Chicken broth (3 c.)

Directions:

1. Bring out a pan and bring the broth to a simmer. When it warms up, take it off the heat.
2. Meanwhile, bring out a big pan and let the oil get warm inside the pot. Throw the onion and barley inside as well and stir it to combine.
3. Turn the heat down and then stir so the onion turns softer and the barley is toasted for five minutes.
4. Add a third of the broth and bring this to a simmer and cook for another 12 minutes until it is absorbed.
5. Repeat with some more broth, slowly adding in the rest of the broth. Your cooking time will be about 50 minutes total.
6. Take the pan off the hit and stir in the pepper, salt, and Parmesan. Serve this warm.

Sweet Potato Chips

Ingredients:

Pepper
Salt
Italian seasoning (1 Tbsp.)
Olive oil (2 tsp.)
Sweet potatoes, sliced (2 lbs.)

Directions:

1. Bring out a big bowl and toss the potatoes together with the pepper, salt, Italian seasoning, and oil.
2. Spread out a bit of this onto a baking sheet and turn the oven on to 400 degrees.
3. Bake the chips for 10 minutes and then use a spatula to turn them over and cooking another 7 minutes. Serve these warm.

Chapter 6: Recipes for Phase 3 of the South Beach Diet

Classic Burger

Ingredients:

Sliced red onion (1/2)
Sliced tomatoes (1/2)
Lettuce (4 leaves)
Dijon mustard (2 tsp.)
Swiss cheese (2 slices)
Pepper (1/4 tsp.)
Salt
Ground beef (3/4 lbs.)

Directions:

1. Heat up a grill and let it be warm. Bring out a container and allow the beef to mix together with some pepper and salt and then mold into patties.
2. Grill the patties until they are done as much as you would like. Layer on the cheese slices and cook for another minute to allow the cheese to melt.
3. Take two leaves of lettuce and layer on different plates and then the patties. Spread the mustard on top and before topping with the onions, tomatoes, and lettuce before serving.

Steak Wraps

Ingredients:

Whole wheat wraps (4)
Salt (1/4 tsp.)
Lime juice (2 tsp.)
Sour cream (1 Tbsp.)
Chopped tomatoes (2)
Romaine lettuce leaves (2)
Flank steak (1 ¼ lb.)
Peppers (1 Tbsp.)

Directions:

1. Take the peppers and rub them all over the steak. Place this into a bag and let it marinate for about an hour.
2. Turn on the broiler and then place the steak inside to cook for 5 minutes on both sides. Take the steak out and let it cool on a cutting board for 5 minutes. Cut into slices.
3. Take out a bowl and combine the salt, lime juice, sour cream, tomatoes, and lettuce.
4. Warm up the wraps in the microwave for 30 seconds and then lay them out. Add the steak and the rest of the ingredients and then roll up tight to finish.

Chili

Ingredients:

Black peppercorns
Salt
Red kidney beans (15 oz.)
Diced tomatoes (28 oz.)
Onion (1)
Cumin (1 tsp.)
Chili powder (2 1/2)
Ground beef (1 lb.)
Olive oil (1 Tbsp.)

Directions:

1. Bring out a pan and heat it up with oil. Add the cumin, a bit of chili powder, and the beef. Cook these for 5 minutes until they are browned.
2. Scoop this onto a plate and then reduce the heat. Fill up an empty saucepan with the rest of the chili powder, the garlic, and the onion.
3. Cook this mixture for 3 minutes to soften the onion before adding the beans and the tomatoes.
4. Cover this up and let it simmer for 10 minutes, stirring a few times. Now add in the beef and let it cook for five more minutes before serving.

Egg Burritos

Ingredients:

Salsa
Sour cream
Cheddar cheese (1 c.)
Tortillas (5)
Spike seasoning (1 tsp.)
Olive oil (1 Tbsp.)
Green chilies (1/2 can)
Green pepper (1/2 diced)
Diced red bell pepper (1/2)
Eggs (6)

Directions:

1. Heat up a pan using some olive oil. Add in both the diced peppers and cook for 4 minutes.
2. Once these are soft, add in the chiles and the spike seasoning and cook for another 2 minutes.
3. While these are cooking, whisk the eggs inside a bowl. Add some oil to the pan and then pour the eggs over the peppers. Cook these until the eggs just start to set.
4. Warm up the tortillas and then place a bit of the peppers and eggs in the middle. Add some cheese, salsa, and sour cream as well.
5. Fold these together and serve right away.

Blackberry Smoothie

Ingredients:

Wheat germ (1 Tbsp.)
Sugar substitute (1 Tbsp.)
Plain yogurt (1 ½ c.)
Blackberries (1 c.)
Banana (2)

Directions:

1. Take out the blender and combine the blackberries and bananas together on the puree setting.
2. Add in the wheat germ, sugar, and yogurt along with some ice cubes and puree a few more minutes.
3. Pour it out and enjoy.

Spiced Apricot Oatmeal

Ingredients:

Salt
Cinnamon (1/2 tsp.)
Maple syrup (1 ½ tsp.)
Dried apricots (12)
Oats (1/2 c.)
Walnuts (1/4 c.)

Directions:

1. Heat up the toaster oven to 275 degrees. Spread the walnuts out on a tray and bake them up for 9 minutes before chopping.
2. Combine together the salt, cinnamon, syrup, apricots, oats, and 2 cups of water and place into a bowl. Cover with some plastic wrap.
3. Cook this for 6 minutes. Stir the oatmeal at this time and then replace the plastic wrap. Cook for 6 more minutes.
4. Add some nuts on the top and serve.

Deviled Eggs

Ingredients:

Smoked paprika
Parsley (2 tsp.)
Salt
Mustard (1/2 tsp.)
Mayo (2 Tbsp.0
Boiled eggs (4)

Directions:

1. Take the eggs and cut them lengthwise to take out the yolks. Take these and place into the food processor.
2. Add in all the ingredients besides the paprika and then puree to make smooth and creamy.
3. Place this mixture into a pastry bag and pipe into the egg white halves. Add the paprika on top and then serve chilled in the fridge.

Fruity Yogurt

Ingredients:

Yogurt (1 c.)
Chilled strawberries (1 handful)
Blueberries (1 handful)

Directions:

1. Take the blueberries and cut them into small pieces. Smash them a bit at the bottom of a bowl.
2. Pour the yogurt over the blueberries but don't mix them.
3. Slice up the strawberries and place them on top of the yogurt, mixing a bit but not enough to get the blueberries.
4. Eat this right away.

Turkey Rolls

Ingredients:

Swiss cheese (6 oz.)
Turkey slices (1 box)
Chives (1/4 c.)
Pepper
Lemon juice (1 Tbsp.)
Lemon zest (1 tsp.)
Yogurt (2 Tbsp.)
Avocado (1/2)

Directions:

1. To start, take the avocado and scoop the innards out. Mash with a potato masher.
2. Mix in the black pepper, salt, lemon juice, and zest.
3. Flatten out some turkey and spread a bit of this all over it. Roll up the slice.
4. Repeat these until the spread is all done and enjoy.

Conclusion

Thank for making it through to the end of *South Beach Diet: Beginners Guide to the South Beach Diet—How to Effectively Lose Weight, Feel Great and Healthy with the South Beach Diet*, let's hope it was informative and able to provide you with all of the tools you need to achieve your goals whatever it may be.

The next step is to get started on this diet plan. We spent some time talking about the different phases that are involved in this diet plan (remember that there are three to help you learn how to lose weight and keep it off) and you will be able to get started with the first one as soon as you are ready to get started. Then you can move through the rest of the phases at your own rate, depending on how much weight you have to lose and how quickly it comes off.

The ideas behind the South Beach Diet are simple and they are there to help you to lose weight efficiently, but you still have to put in some of the work. This is not a quick plan that will be easy and you can lose weight in your sleep, but if you follow the advice that is in this guidebook and use some of these recipes to help you out, you will find that losing weight can be easier than ever before. When you are ready to finally lose that weight that has been sticking around for years, make sure to pick up this guidebook and learn about the South Beach Diet.

Finally, if you found this book useful in anyway, a review on Amazon is always appreciated!

Description

The South Beach Diet is one of the best diet plans that you can choose to go on when you finally want to kick all those bad habits to the curb and lose weight. Many times the hardest part about losing weight is all those cravings that make you go back to your old habits in no time. The South Beach Diet is meant to help you get through some of these issues so that you can lose weight and keep it off for good.

This guidebook is going to spend some time talking about the South Beach Diet and how it can help you to finally lose the weight. Some of the things that you will learn about this diet plan include:

What is the South Beach Diet?
The truth about how carbs work in the body.
The 3 Phases of the South Beach Diet and how to eat right on each of them.
Recipes to use during each phase of this diet plan.

When you are ready to start losing weight and feeling better without all those cravings driving you nuts, it is time to learn about the South Beach Diet and how it can improve your life and make losing weight easier.

www.ingramcontent.com/pod-product-compliance
Lightning Source LLC
Chambersburg PA
CBHW071254280526
45788CB00004B/1716